Effective Guide and Cookbook for Autism and ADHD In Children

Including best 50 autism-friendly recipes, mealtime tips and exercises; to help improve your child's condition

@ Dr. Sam Ludington

All rights reserved. No parts of this publication may be reproduced, stored in retrieval system, or transmitted in any form or by any means, electronic, mechanical, photocopying, recording, or otherwise, without the prior written permission of the author.

Contents

iv

Introduction

Autism, also known as autism spectrum disorder (ASD), is a complex disease that includes communication and behavior problems. It may involve multiple symptoms and skills. ASD can be a minor problem, or it can be a disability that requires full-time care in a special facility. Autism, sometimes called autism spectrum disorder (ASD), is a lifelong disease that affects how a person experiences the world around them, how they communicate and interact socially, including their interests and behavior.

It is called the "spectrum disorder" because it can affect people in different ways and to different degrees. This is also a kind of "hidden disability" because people usually cannot tell from the outside that someone has autism. It is difficult for them to understand the thoughts and feelings of others. This makes it difficult for them to express themselves with words or gestures, facial expressions and touch. People with autism often have difficulty in learning. Their learning skills may improve in an unusual manner. For instance, they may have trouble communicating, but they are exceptionally good at art, music, mathematics or memory. Therefore, they may perform particularly well in analysis or problem-solving tests.

Now, more children are diagnosed with autism than ever before. But the latest number may be higher because of changes in the way it is diagnosed, not because there are more children suffering from the disease. The disease affects approximately 700,000 people in the UK, more than 1 in 100 people. It is becoming more and more common throughout the world, and people with autism often suffer from stigma, discrimination and human rights violations. Although some symptoms may vary from person to person, it is important that once you discover your child's symptoms, you should seek medical help immediately.

Read on to know more about the disorder, which includes the forms, symptoms in children and how to diagnose the disease.

Types of Autism Spectrum Disorders

These types were once thought to be separate conditions. Now, they fall under the range of autism spectrum disorders. They include:

Asperger's syndrome: These children have no language problems. In fact, their scores on intelligence tests are often in the average or above-average range. But they have social problems and apathy.

Autistic Disorder: this is what comes to people's minds when they hear the word "autism". It refers to issues with social contact, interaction, and gaming in children under the age of three.

Childhood Disintegrative Disorder: For at least two years, these children grow normally, but then lose some or all of their speech and social skills.

Pervasive developmental disorder (PDD or atypical autism): If your child exhibits some autistic behavior, such as difficulties in social and communication skills, but does not fit into another category, your doctor may use this phrase.

Causes of ASD

The exact cause of autism is unknown. Problems in the parts of your brain that perceive sensory feedback and process language may be to blame.

Boys are four times more likely than girls to have autism. It may affect people of any race, ethnicity, or socioeconomic status. A child's risk of autism is unaffected by family income, lifestyle, or educational level. Since autism runs in families, some genetic combinations can increase a child's risk.

Autism is more likely in a child who has an older parent.

Pregnant mothers who are exposed to certain substances or chemicals during their pregnancy, such as liquor or anti-seizure medications, are more likely to give birth to autistic children. Maternal metabolic disorders such as diabetes and obesity are also risk factors. Autism has also been attributed to untreated phenylketonuria (also known as PKU, a metabolic condition caused by an enzyme deficiency) and rubella (German measles).

In addition, there is no proof that vaccines cause autism. People would understand more of the habits affected by the disorder if they are educated about it.

Autism Signs and Symptoms

Autism symptoms normally begin before a child reaches the age of three. Some people exhibit symptoms from the moment they are born. The following are some of the most common autism symptoms:

- Inability to make eye contact.
- A limited range of interests or a strong desire to learn more about a specific subject.
- Repeating something, such as repeating words or sentences, pacing back and forth, or turning a lever, over and over.

- High sensitivity to sounds, touches, smells, or sights that other people consider normal.
- Not staring at or paying attention to other persons.
- When someone points something out to you, you don't look at it.
- Reluctance to be kissed or cuddled.

- Speech, gestures, facial expressions, or voice tone are difficult to understand or use.
- Using a sing-song, flat, or robotic tone of voice.
- Difficulty in adapting to routine changes Some children with autism may also have seizures. These may not start until puberty.

Signs of Autism in Babies and Toddlers

There are several signs that children have autism, mainly related to their ways of communication and interaction. If you notice any of these early symptoms in your baby or toddler, please see your general practitioner or health care. Preschool children with autism may experience the following symptoms:

- Speech production is delayed or nonexistent.
- Refusing to accept cuddles from a parent or guardian (they may prefer to initiate cuddles themselves)
- When they're asked to do something, they show a negative reaction.
- Insensitivity to people invading their own personal space or a lack of knowledge of other people's personal space
- Prefer to play alone and have no interest in playing with other age mates.
- When talking, gestures and facial expressions are seldom used.
- Face contact is avoided at all costs.
- Swaying back and forth, for example (repetitive movement).
- Playing with toys in a monotonous, unimaginative manner

- Preference for familiar routines and irritability when the routine is changed
- Having a strong dislike for certain foods because of their texture, color, or flavor
- Unusual sensory interests – children with ASD, for example, can improperly sniff toys, objects, or people.
- Despite having normal hearing, they do not answer when their name is called.

Signs of Autism in Teenagers

School-aged children with autism can exhibit the following symptoms in addition to the ones mentioned above:

- Avoiding the use of spoken language is a preference.
- Monotonous voice, with a preference for pre-learned phrases at times
- Two-way conversations are difficult, and you may seem to be talking 'at' people.
- Understanding things literally and being unable to understand sarcasm, metaphors or figures of speech

- Not being aware of certain simple social interactions.

Diagnosing for ASD

Autism is typically diagnosed in children around the age of two, according to the NHS. This is when the condition's main symptoms, such as social contact and engagement, begin to manifest, and others only become apparent when the child's routine changes, such as beginning nursery or school.

If your child has some of the symptoms of autism, the first step in finding a diagnosis is to see your doctor or health visitor. Other practitioners can be referred to you, such as a psychologist, psychiatrist, pediatrician, or physiotherapist.

Treating autism

While there is no 'specific cure' for autism, an official diagnosis will help children receive the treatment and support they need.

As the disease affects individuals differently, there are different approaches to supporting children. SPELL, TEACCH, Social Stories, and counseling are some of the most popular, but the best option would depend on the circumstances.

According to the National Autistic Society, every approach to assisting a child with autism should be constructive, focusing on the child's strengths and assisting them in realizing their full potential while also growing encouragement.

FACTS TO KNOW ABOUT AUTISM SPECTRUM DISORDER

o Though the word "autism" was coined in 1911, until the late twentieth century, little was understood or medically studied about autism spectrum disorder.

> Today, new discoveries and developments are being made to help people on the spectrum reach their full potential.

o Autism now affects one out of every 100 children. ASD is diagnosed almost 5 times more often in boys than in children.

o In the United States, autism spectrum disorder is one of the fastest-growing psychological disorders. ASD is more prevalent than cancer, diabetes, and AIDS combined in children.

o Autism is derived from the Greek word autos, which means "self." It literally means "alone."

- o Autism spectrum disorder affects people of all races, creeds, and sects, as well as people of both sexes. It doesn't discriminate or influence one party over the other.

- o Autism spectrum disorder (ASD) is a form of developmental condition that usually manifests before the age of three.

- o It is preferable to diagnose and treat autism spectrum disorder as soon as possible. Early diagnosis and care have a huge impact on the lives of children.

- o Although the causes of ASD are unknown, it is understood that parental activity prior to, during, and after pregnancy does not contribute to the development of ASD.

- o Autism spectrum disorder patients have communication problems. It's important to differentiate between lack of spoken language and lack of social contact.

- o Being nonverbal at age 4 does not imply autistic children will never speak.

According to studies, the majority of people will learn to use vocabulary, and almost half will learn to speak fluently.

o Adults and children with autism spectrum disorder also have a strong desire to help others, but they lack the capacity to develop empathic and socially linked normal actions on their own. Individuals with ASD often want to socialize, but they lack the opportunity to acquire successful social skills on their own.

o If one identical twin has autism spectrum disorder, the other twin has a 60-96 percent risk of having ASD as well. While fraternal twins have a lower risk of both getting ASD, if one has an ASD the other has up to a 24 percent likelihood.

o Allergies, asthma, seizures, digestive disorders, eating disorders, sleeping disorders, sensory processing dysfunction, cognitive impairments, and other medical disorders are common comorbid medical conditions in autism spectrum disorder.

o Seizures affect up to a third of people with autism spectrum disorder; the incidence of seizures in people with ASD is ten times higher than the general population.

o A genetic, neurological, or metabolic disorder affects about 10% of children with autism spectrum disorder.

o Children and adults with ASD have the ability to communicate and connect with others. They may be making good eye contact. They may be either verbal or nonverbal. They may be very bright, average in intellect, or suffer from cognitive impairment.

o Autism spectrum disorder is often associated with hyperlexia, or the ability to read above one's age or grade level in school.

o Individuals with autism spectrum disorder can be very artistic, and they can quickly develop a passion and talent for music, theatre, painting, dancing, and singing.

o Albert Einstein, Isaac Newton, Andy Warhol, and Bill Gates are all stated to be on the autism spectrum.

o Females with autism spectrum disorder are indeed understudied in the scientific community.

o Many individuals with autism spectrum disorder are living successfully, happily, contributing to the well-being of their families and others. When appropriate services are provided during the child's educational years, this is most likely to occur.

DEVELOPMENTAL SCREENINGS FOR ASD
According to the American Academy of Pediatrics (AAP), all babies should be screened for ASD between the ages of 18 and 24 months, Early detection of children who may have ASD may be aided by screening. Early detection and intervention can be beneficial to these children.

It's important to remember that screening is not the same as a diagnosis. Children who test positive for ASD do not always have the condition. Furthermore, scans do not always detect every child with ASD.

Other screenings and tests

Your child's GP may recommend a combination of tests for autism, such as:

- Checking for genetic diseases using DNA
  • Behavioral assessment
- Visual and auditory assessments to rule out any visual or hearing problems that aren't caused by autism.
- Autism Diagnostic Observation Schedule and other developmental questionnaires
  (ADOS)

- A team of experts usually makes the diagnosis. Child psychologists, occupational therapists, and speech and language pathologists may be part of this team.

While there are no "cure" options for autism, therapy and other treatment options can help people feel better and reduce their symptoms.

- Many treatment options include treatments like:
- Behavioral therapy is a type of counseling that focuses on
- Play therapy
- Occupational therapy
- Physical therapy
- Speech therapy

Alternative treatments for improving autism may include:

- High-dose vitamins
- Chelation therapy, which involves flushing metals from the system
- Hyperbaric oxygen therapy
- Melatonin to tackle insomnia

Note: Some of these treatments can be harmful.

ADHD and Autism

Attention deficit hyperactivity disorder (ADHD) and autism may be similar to each other. Children with either disorder may have trouble concentrating. They can be emotionally unstable or have a hard time interacting. They can struggle with schoolwork and interpersonal relationships.

Despite the fact that they have many of the same symptoms, the two conditions are not the same. Autism spectrum disorders are a form of developmental disorders that affect language, behavior, social interactions, and learning abilities. ADHD has an impact on how the brain grows and evolves. One can have both.

The correct diagnosis early on helps children get the right treatment so they don't miss out on important development and learning. People with these conditions can have successful, happy lives.

Keep an eye on how your child pays attention. Those with autism struggle to focus on things that they don't like, such as reading a book or doing a puzzle. And they may fixate on things that they do like, such as playing with a particular toy. Kids with ADHD dislike and avoid things they'll have to concentrate on.

Making the right diagnosis as early as possible helps children get the right treatment, so as to avoid missing important development and learning opportunities. These people can live good and happy lives despite their circumstances.

Differences between autism and ADHD

Keep an eye on how attentive your child is. Autism makes it difficult for kids to concentrate on something they don't like, such as reading a book or solving a puzzle. They can even become obsessed on things they love, such as playing with a specific toy. Things that demand attention are disliked and avoided by children with ADHD.

You should also examine how your child is developing communication skills. Although both conditions make it difficult for children to communicate with others, children with autism have a lower level of social awareness. They often have trouble putting their thoughts and feelings into words, and they may not be able to point to an object to give their speech meaning.

It is difficult for them to maintain eye contact.

On the other hand, a child with ADHD can talk nonstop. They're more likely to jump in and dominate a conversation while someone else is speaking. Consider the subject as well. Some autistic children can talk for hours about a topic that interests them. While an autistic child enjoys order and repetition, an ADHD child does not, even if it is favorable to them. For example, a child with autism can crave the same food at a favorite restaurant or become excessively attached to a single toy or shirt. When routines are disrupted, they will become agitated. A kid with ADHD dislikes doing the same thing over and over again for long periods of time.

Diagnosis

If you suspect your child has ADHD or autism, consult your doctor on the appropriate tests. There is no single test that can decide if a child has either or both of these conditions. You can begin by consulting your pediatrician, who will refer you to a specialist.

Doctors search for a pattern of habits such as being distracted or forgetful, not following through, having difficulty waiting for a turn, and fidgeting or squirming. Parents, teachers, and other people who care about the child will be asked for input. Other potential causes of the symptoms would be ruled out by a doctor. A parent's response to a questionnaire about their child, mostly about behaviors that began when they were very young, is the first step in getting an autism diagnosis. More questionnaires, surveys, and checklists, as well as interviews and observed behaviors, may be used in future studies and resources.

Note: It's also possible for a person to have both autism and ADHD.

Impact of diet on autism
There isn't a specific diet for people with ASD Despite these challenges, some autism experts are looking at dietary modifications to deal with behavioral problems and overall quality of life.

A basis of the autism diet is the elimination of artificial additives. Preservatives, colors, and sweeteners are among them.

Instead, an autism diet should concentrate on whole foods like:

- Fresh fruits and vegetables
- Lean poultry
- Fish
- Unsaturated fats
- Lots of water

A gluten-free diet is also recommended by some autism experts. Wheat, barley, and other grains all contain the protein gluten.

Diet is important improve symptoms of attention-deficit hyperactivity disorder (ADHD), a condition related to autism, according to some studies and anecdotal evidence.

PHYSICAL ACTIVITIES FOR KIDS WITH AUTISM

Certain activities can help children with autism manage their frustrations and improve their overall well-being.

Every sort of physical activity that your child likes is beneficial. Walking and actually enjoying a good time on the playground are also excellent options.

Swimming and being in the water can be used for exercise as well as sensory play. Sensory play games can help people with autism who have difficulty processing sensory signals.

For children with autism, touch sports can be challenging at times. Other types of difficult yet strengthening exercises can be recommended instead. Start with these autism exercises for kids, such as arm circles and star jumps.

Important Exercises for Kids with Autism

Studies suggest that physical exercise lasting longer than 20 minutes can help children with autism reduce stereotypical behaviors, hyperactivity, and hostility. Exercise not only helps children with autism participate more fully with their surroundings, but it also aids weight loss and improves overall health.

For kids with autism, full-body workouts are the perfect way to improve balance, stamina, endurance, and body knowledge. Here are five exercises to get you started.

Tips for getting started

It's important to teach a new activity to a child with autism in a relaxed and welcoming atmosphere. Use phrases like "You're doing a fantastic job!" as positive reinforcement. Using verbal or physical prompts to direct them through the gestures and reduce the likelihood of them being irritated or upset.

Crawling Bears

Bear crawls help with body awareness, balance, and motor planning, as well as trunk and upper body strength.

Begin by kneeling on your hands and knees, with your hands under your shoulders and your knees under your hips.

Extend your legs to the point where they are slightly bent. Spread your fingers wide to get the best grip on the floor.

Walk about 10-20 feet around the floor with your feet and hands.

Keep this posture and walk backwards in the same manner.

For best results, try varying the speed and direction. If this action is too difficult, an instructor should provide hands-on assistance at the hips.

Medicine Ball Slams
Throwing heavy balls like medicine balls will enhance core strength and balance and actually boost coordination. It may also have medicinal effects and may activate parts of the brain responsible for short-term memory.

Begin in a standing posture with both hands holding a medicine ball.

Lift the ball with straight arms above your head.

With as much energy as possible, throw the ball to the turf.

Pick up the ball by bending your knees and repeat the movement 20 times.

You can make this activity more difficult by tossing the ball at a target or increasing the ball's weight.

Star Jumps

Jumping activities are excellent full-body workouts that enhance cardiorespiratory fitness, leg and core strength, and body awareness. Star jumps can be done one at a time or in several repetitions and can be practiced anywhere.

Squat down with your knees bent, feet flat on the floor, and arms tucked in toward your stomach.

Quickly rise from squatting and form an X with your arms and legs.

Return to starting place with arms and legs tucked in after landing. Repeat for up to 20 reps or until you're exhausted.

Arm Circles

The authors of a study published in Research in Autism Spectrum Disorders discovered that movements similar to those seen in people with autism may help provide the body with required feedback. This can help to minimize repetitive activities like flapping arms or clapping. Arm circles are a perfect upper-body workout that can be performed anywhere with no equipment and helps improve flexibility and strength in the shoulders and back.

Standing with your feet shoulder-width apart and your arms at your sides, stand tall.

At shoulder height, extend your arms straight out to the side.

Make tiny circles with your hands while holding your arms straight.

Make the circles larger and larger as you go, generating movement from the shoulders.

Repeat 20 times in one direction, then in the opposite direction.

Mirror Exercises

Autism is characterized by difficulties communicating with others and interacting with the world. Mirror drills enable children to imitate what they see others doing, which can improve balance, body awareness, and social skills.

Stand with your hands by your side, facing a partner.

Begin by making slow arm movements with your partner. Start with circles and work your way up to more complicated patterns.

When you're confident, imitate your partner's movements as if you were looking in the mirror. If they lift their right arm, for example, you raise your left arm.

To get more feedback, gently touch your palms.

Continue doing this for another 1-2 minutes. Other body pieces, such as the head, trunk, and legs, may be used. Rep 3-5 times more.

Advice from the experts

Before beginning an exercise regimen for a child with autism, always consult a doctor.

- Start slowly and keep an eye alert for signs of exhaustion, such as shortness of breath, muscle cramps, or dizziness.
- Before exercising, make sure the child is properly hydrated and rested.
- It's best to begin with a low intensity and gradually increase to harder, more strenuous sessions.

MEALTIME TIPS FOR AUTISTIC CHILDREN WITH EATING CHALLENGES

A therapist from the Autism Speaks Autism Treatment Network shares some tips for bettering nutrition and mealtime activity.

Feeding difficulties are one of the most common concerns that parents and children with autism bring to the table.

Of course, parents all over the world are concerned about their children's nutrition and mealtime activity. However, evidence backs up that children with autism are much more likely to be particularly picky about what they eat. As a result, their diets are often less varied than those of their normally developing siblings and mates.

In this article, I'm excited to share some of the techniques that have proven to be the most effective in assisting children and their families in developing healthier eating habits in my experience. Keep in mind that it's a path that mostly includes setbacks as well as triumphs.

Rule out physical problems.

It is common for children with autism to have medical problems that make eating unpleasant. These may include tooth decay, difficulty chewing and painful acid reflux. Therefore, before proceeding, make sure your child's doctor screens and resolves any such issues.

Ease into mealtime

As the meal time approaches, many children with autism will feel great anxiety. The root causes may include feeling aversion and fear of unfamiliar food. Inadvertently, the family may try to force the child to eat, thereby forming a pattern of tight meal times, which intensifies anxiety. Fear and anxiety will put the child's body in a state of fighting or flight, thereby effectively eliminating hunger.

To resolve this situation, it is suggested that parents and other caregivers take a few minutes to help their children relax before eating. One way is to practice deep breathing together for five minutes. This can be very simple, for example, slowly and deeply inhale as four, and then slowly and completely inhale as seven or eight. In addition, the two of you can blow pinwheels, bubbles or even wind instruments, such as tape recorders or harmonicas.

You might also spend those five minutes performing a "deep pressure tactile exercise," which involves pressing your hands against a wall (leaning in with your full weight) or making your child press his or her palms against yours.

Sit together at a table for meals

I can't stress enough how important it is for a family to eat together on a regular basis. Environmental cues assist all children, especially those with autism, in learning what they should be doing. A child's bed, for example, is an environmental signal for sleeping. Similarly, the family table should be used to feed.

Furthermore, eating with your child encourages learning through emulation. Children are biologically programmed to imitate what they see. And if a child sees you putting new foods in your mouth, he or she is more likely to do so as well.

Sometimes, the first move is to eliminate bad habits like eating in front of the TV, sitting on a parent's lap, playing with a touch screen, and so on. Parents should begin by having their kids sit at the table with them or another family member, even if only for a minute. Gradually increase the time at the table to around 20 minutes with praise and small rewards.

Reassure your child that eating isn't required at first. To further guide your child where to sit and what to expect, I recommend using the same table for all meals and having family members sit in the same chairs.

Support your child's posture

The core muscles of the stomach and back are often weak in autistic children. Others lack awareness of their own bodies. That is, they have a hard time determining where their bodies are in space. While sitting at the dinner table, all of these issues can cause poor posture, wriggling, and discomfort. You will help your child concentrate on eating rather than holding his or her body on the chair by offering encouragement

If your child is slouching, leaning, or wriggling at the table, wrap rolled towels around his or her back and hips for added support. Make sure the feet are supported as well. Place a step stool in front of the chair and under the table if they can't reach the floor.

Establish acceptance to new foods through gradual exposure

In my experience, I've worked with children who have genuine aversions to some foods. I've noticed that many of these kids have especially strong reactions to the sight of food. Several of the children in my practice, for example, refuse to eat foods of certain colors. Another child is terrified of handling apples because they seem to be "wet." A third child is terrified of even being in the same room as an orange

It's critical to recognize and comprehend that these fears are just as strong as, say, a fear of snakes or large spiders. With this in mind, I begin to use incremental exposure concepts to assist them in learning to control and eventually eliminate these fears.

Take for instance, the kid who felt uneasy around apples. We started by getting him used to just staring at an apple in front of him for a few minutes. I reassured him that he didn't have to eat it and praised him. We then went on to using a fork, a napkin, and finally his fingers to touch the fruit. We used game-based words, such as "I challenge you to keep the apple to your cheek for 30 seconds." He also learned to chop up the apple in a food processor, all of which helped him conquer what had previously been a very real fear.

Create timetables for meals and stick to them

It's important to eat on a schedule, as discussed previously. Space meals and desserts every twoand-a-half to three hours throughout the day. Snacks, including milk and juice, should be avoided in between. The goal is to associate particular mealtimes with your child's internal hunger signals. This aids your child's body in anticipating and accepting food at scheduled times.

Go stretch your child's favorite meals

Let's say white spaghetti with no sauce is a kid's all-time favorite. Begin by offering a different brand of white pasta, then brown rice or another form of spaghetti to "stretch" his or her food acceptance. You'll eventually progress to spaghetti with a little butter, then a white sauce, and so on. The goal is to provide a food that looks familiar while increasing tolerance for tiny, gradual changes. A switch from spaghetti to penne pasta, for example, can be too much to handle simply because the two types of pasta are so distinguishable.

Remove food from their brand boxes

When I hear of children who only eat one brand of a particular food my alarm bells go off. I know a few parents who spend an excessive amount of time looking for specific brands because their children refuse to eat anything else. I advise my clients to stop this problem entirely by removing food from boxes as soon as they unpack their groceries. Put the food in clear containers. To avoid your child being "trapped" on a highly specific flavor, appearance, or texture, rotate products as much as possible.

Allow your child to experiment, play, and get their hands dirty with food

Playing with food is one of the ways that children learn. This ties in well with the concept of "gradual exposure" that I mentioned earlier. Encourage your child to use his or her senses to communicate with food. Discuss the appearance and texture of foods. Use cookie cutters and other tools to create unique shapes.

Consider it "meal school," and set aside some time per week to participate in hands-on food learning. Your child might or might not consume the foods he or she is experimenting with. The aim is to lay a foundation that helps increase food comfort.

Focus on the food rather than your child's behavior.

Try to ignore challenging habits at the table as much as possible. Many children learn to avoid the family meal by spitting, crying, pounding on the table, and other similar behaviors. I recommend talking about food to divert attention away from the negative behavior. This can be accomplished by posing the following questions to engage the entire family in "food learning."

- Is this a canned or dried product?
- Does this food have little or a huge smell?
- What distinguishes this pita bread from regular bread?

- When you chew this food, what sound does it make?
- What other foods do we eat in the same color family?

The Best Foods for Children with Autism: Fatty fish and fortified eggs

These foods all contain the beneficial omega 3 fatty acid. The American diet is deficient in healthy fats, especially omega 3. Omega-3 fatty acids are anti-inflammatory. Autism, dyslexia, ADHD, depression, anxiety, and dyspraxia have all been attributed to a lack of omega 3 fatty acids [1]. While there is no definitive proof that omega 3 supplementation can boost ASD symptoms including language and hyperactivity, there is published and anecdotal evidence that it can. The good news is that having more omega 3 foods in your child's diet would have no negative effects. Omega 3s are mainly present in fatty fish such as salmon, herring, mackerel, and sardines, which makes them difficult to come by. Fortunately, it can also be found in fortified eggs and milder fish like cod and canned tuna. Three times a week, serve free-range omega 3 eggs and fatty fish. For young fish skeptics, fish cakes or burgers, fish sticks, and tacos can be good starting points.

If possible, purchase wild fish. Not only is sustainably raised fish healthier for the ecosystem, but it also contains more nutrients and contains less mercury than farm-raised fish.

Incorporate grass-fed beef and animal proteins from sustainable sources

Guess what? Grass-fed beef is also high in omega 3 fats, which are beneficial to your health. In comparison to conventionally raised beef, grass-fed beef contains more healthy fats, more beneficial nutrients (such as vitamins A and E), and less beneficial nutrients (such as cholesterol). Grass-fed beef, like free-range chicken and other organic animal proteins, has less toxins like hormones and antibiotics. For children with food sensitivities and health problems like autism, this may make a big difference. Since it is a source of B12, animal protein is helpful for children with autism. B12 is essential for the nervous system, according to some research.

Shellfish, beans, nuts, seeds are ideal

Most children on the spectrum have low zinc levels, possibly as a result of their restricted diets. Autism has also been linked to low zinc levels in children, according to research. Zinc is a nutrient that influences taste, in addition to its association with ASD. Picky eating can be cured by increasing zinc levels. Zinc-rich foods, such as shellfish, beef, fortified cereals, beans, peas, yogurt, cheese, cashews, pork, chickpeas, lentils, and almonds, should be consumed on a regular basis.

FOOD SUPPLEMENTS FOR AUTISM

Autistic children may have dietary limitations or preferences. It's also possible that they break down fat in different ways. As a result, such nutrients are often lacking in autistic children. Any of these nutrients have been researched to see whether providing them to children as supplements will help with autism symptoms. More study, however, is required. Consult your child's physician or a dietitian before feeding him or her any of the supplements mentioned below.

Vitamins and Minerals

Multivitamins: According to some studies, taking a multivitamin will help autistic children with sleep and digestive issues. It's worth noting that taking a multivitamin with iron can trigger digestive issues. Giving your child a multivitamin isn't harmful and may even be beneficial, particularly if he or she isn't eating a well-balanced diet.

Iron: Iron deficiency is widespread in children with autism, owing to their picky eating habits. Request that your child's iron levels be tested on a regular basis by his or her doctor. An iron supplement can aid in restoring iron back to normal levels. Unless your kid's iron level has been confirmed as inadequate by a health care provider, do not offer an iron supplement

Omega-3 Fatty Acids: According to some studies, many autistic children have low omega3 fat levels. Omega-3 supplements can benefit autistic children with hyperactivity. Nevertheless, further research is required before omega-3 supplements can be prescribed for autistic children.

The Gluten-Free, Casein-Free Diet

Gluten is the primary protein present in wheat, rye, barley, triticale, kamut, and spelt. Dairy products including cow's milk, cheese, yogurt, and ice cream contain casein as the main protein. This diet could be recommended to help autistic children change their behavior. When adopting this diet, some children with autism experience a short-term reduction in autistic behaviors.

Food-Related Challenges

Autistic children exhibit a wide range of symptoms, including challenging behaviors. As we all know, autism affects each child differently. So, when it comes to food, keep in mind that every child has their own preferences. Here are a few examples:

- Limited food choice

- Foods high in sugar, salt, and/or fat are preferred exclusively.
- Insistence on specific labels, designs, and temperatures.

Routine Meal Schedule

It simply refers to mealtimes. Inconsistent mealtime routines may serve as a deterrent to food consumption. So, as far as possible, aim to adhere to a regular meal schedule. Kids with autism are more likely to participate in positive actions because they have predictable patterns.

Have a Food Diary

Many children with autism use their behaviors to express what they can't say verbally. As a result, keeping track of what your child eats can help you link behavioral symptoms to nutrition. You'll be able to spot trends and patterns more easily as you go. This will eventually lead you to the type of diet that is best for you.

AUTISM-FRIENDLY RECIPES FOR YOUR KIDS AND FAMILY

So, without further ado, here are some recipes!

Gluten-Free Autism Recipes

Gluten-free dieting is quite difficult in today's world, given that so many foods have it. But it does have a huge benefit. In a gluten-free diet, you'll be replacing all gluten products with ricebased alternatives. Rice bread, rice noodles, and rice cakes are a few examples. Certain corn products are also labeled as gluten-free. However, be careful as corn products have several risks.

Pork Chops with Carrots and Toasted Buckwheat

Prep Time: 30 Minutes

Cook Time: 25 Minutes

Servings: 4

Ingredients

- 1 orange
- 1 garlic clove well grated
- kosher salt
- 2 tablespoons olive oil
- 1½ pound carrots, scrubbed, halved lengthwise, cut into 2 pieces
- 2 teaspoons fresh lime juice, plus more
- ¾ cup pearled buckwheat groats
- 1 tablespoon vegetable oil
- 2 1"-thick bone-in pork shoulder chops (about 8–10 oz. each)
- 3 tablespoons unsalted butter, divided ¼ cup dill sprigs
- Aleppo or Urfa pepper or ground red pepper flakes

Preparation

Step 1

Remove the orange's peel and white pith, dispose. Cut along the sides of membranes to release segments over a small bowl; squeeze in juice as well.

Step 2

Preheat the oven to 450°. On a rimmed baking sheet, combine the carrots, garlic, and 2 tablespoons of olive oil; season with salt. Roast, tossing once in a while, for 15–20 minutes, or until tender and golden brown. While the carrot mixture is still hot, insert orange portions and juice and 2 tsp. lime juice and stir to coat. Set aside.

Step 3

Boil the buckwheat in a large saucepan of hot salted water until tender but not dissolved, for 10–15 minutes. Rinse with cold water after draining. Place on a baking sheet and set aside to dry. **Step 4**

In a large heavy skillet, heat the vegetable oil on high heat. Season the pork with salt and cook for 4 minutes per side, or until browned but still pink in the center. With 1 tbsp. butter, spooned over chops, fry for 1 minute, turning once.

Switch to the cutting board and let it settle for 10 minutes.

Step 5

In the meantime, add the cooled buckwheat and the remaining 2 Tbsp. butter to skillet; sprinkle with salt. Cook, stirring frequently, until the grains are toasted and some are crisp, around 5 minutes. Drain on paper towels.

Step 6

Slice the pork; pour the dill into the buckwheat. Serve the toasted buckwheat and carrots with pork slices, drizzle with lime juice and olive oil and top with Aleppo pepper.

Bacon Pimento Cheese Dip

Prep Time: 10 Minutes

Cook Time: 25 Minutes

Servings: 7

Ingredients

- 4 ounces cream cheese

- 8 slices jones dairy farm dry aged bacon
- 1 cup mayonnaise

- 2-3 scallions shredded
- 1 4oz jar pimentos thinly sliced, drained
- 2 jalapeno peppers seeded and thinly sliced
- salt and pepper to taste
- 2 cups cheddar cheese shredded, extra sharp
- 2 cups pepper jack cheese shredded

Preparation

Step 1

Put the bacon in a large deep-frying pan over medium heat until crispy. Transfer it to paper towels and crumble.

Step 2

In a medium bowl, whisk together bacon, mayonnaise, cream cheese, allspice, jalapenos, green onions, and shredded cheese. Season with salt and pepper.

Step 3

Spread the mixture evenly into a 2-quart casserole and bake for 25 minutes or until the cheese is completely melted and frothy.

<u>**Nutrition Facts Per Serving**</u>

Calories 201 |**Total Fat** 18g |

Sodium 342mg |**Total Carb.** 2g |**Sugars** 1g |**Protein** 7g

Bacon Wrapped Pineapple Bites

Prep Time: 15 minutes

Cook Time: 30 minutes

Servings: 20

Ingredients

- 2 tablespoons honey
- 1-pound bacon slices

- 1 20 ounce can dole pineapple chunks well drained

- ¼-1/2 teaspoon chipotle chile powder
- 1 tablespoon green onion finely sliced, for garnish (optional)

Preparation

Step 1

Preheat the oven to 400°F. Line the sheet pan with the foil and place the wire rack on top of it. Each bacon strip should be cut in half.

Step 2

By skewering one end of a bacon strip, then the pineapple, wrap three pineapple chunks in bacon. Wrap one side of the pineapple chunk in bacon and skewer the middle part of the bacon strip. Another pineapple chunk is skewered, then the bacon is folded over one side of the pineapple. Add a third pineapple chunk to the skewer.

Step 3

Drizzle honey over the bites and gently dust with chipotle Chile powder.

Step 4

Bake for 30 minutes, or until bacon is crisp, flipping each skewer halfway through. If needed, garnish with green onion.

Baked Spaghetti Squash Carbonara

Prep Time: 1 hour

Cook Time: 1 hour

Servings: 10

Ingredients

- 1 medium spaghetti squash approx. 3 pounds
- 1 teaspoon salt
- 4 large eggs
- 8 ounces jones dairy farm bacon 8-10 slices, chopped
- 1 small yellow onion diced
- ½ cup ricotta cheese
- 1 ¼ cups parmesan cheese
- 1 teaspoon black pepper

Preparation

Step 1

Heat the oven to 350°F.

Step 2

Using a sharp kitchen knife, cut the squash in half lengthwise. With a spoon, pick out the seeds and seed flesh and dispose.

Step 3

Place the squash cut-side down in a 9-x13-inch baking dish filled with ½ cup water. Roast for 45 minutes, or until tender.

Step 4

Cook the bacon in a heavy skillet over medium heat until the edges are crisp. Cook for 5 to 6 minutes, or until they are soft and lightly browned. Take off the heat.

Step 5

Whisk the eggs in a big pan, then add the ricotta. Fold in the cooked bacon, onions, 1 cup grated cheese, salt and pepper.

Step 6

Remove the squash from the oven when it can easily be pierced with a fork and increase the temperature to 375°F.

Step 7

Allow the squash to cool slightly after removing it from the baking dish.

Step 8

Remove any remaining water from the baking dish, wipe it dry, and gently grease it with cooking spray.

Step 9

Remove the outer shell of the squash and shred the inside into spaghetti-like strings with a fork. It should be over 6 cups total.

Step 10

In a mixing bowl, combine the squash strings and the egg-and-onion mixture.

Step 11

Place the mixture in the baking dish and top with the unused ¼ cup of cheese. Bake for 45 minutes, or until the top is firm and golden.

Nutrition Facts Per Serving

Calories 166 |**Total Fat** 9g **Sodium** 761mg |**Potassium** 175mg
Total Carb. 8g |**Dietary Fiber** 1g |Sugars 3g |**Protein** 12g

Peach Clouds

This is a simple but elegant dessert. It should be scheduled at least 8 hours in advance, but it is well worth the time. Serve with a scoop of vanilla ice cream on the side. Serve with edible flowers or mint leaves as a garnish. Elegant is an understatement.

Prep Time: 20 minutes

Cook Time: 8 hours **Servings:**

Ingredients

- ¼ teaspoon salt

- 7 egg whites
- 1 teaspoon vanilla extract
- ½ teaspoon cream of tartar
- 1 ½ cups white sugar
- 6 fresh peaches (peeled, pitted, and diced)

Preparation

Step 1

Preheat the oven to 450 degrees F.

Step 2

In a clean, dry bowl, beat egg whites for 2 minutes with an electric mixer. Combine the salt and cream of tartar in the mixing bowl. Continue to beat and add a few tablespoons of sugar at a time until the mixture is glossy and stiff peaks shape. Fold in the vanilla extract.

Step 3

Spoon or pipe into a greased pie plate or onto parchment-lined baking sheets.

Step 4

Place in preheated oven and switch oven off. Leave the meringue in the oven closed, for 8 hours or overnight. To serve, arrange peaches on top of the meringue on a serving platter.

Crispy Apple-Oat Fritters

If the batter thickens as it sits, soften with more club soda.

Prep Time: 20 minutes

Cook Time: 30 minutes

Servings: 8

Ingredients

- 1 large egg
- ½ cup rice flour
- ½ cup (or more) club soda
- ½ cup plus 2 tbsp. sugar, separated
- 1½ teaspoon ground cinnamon, separated
- vegetable oil (for frying; about 4 cups)

- 1 cup gluten-free old-fashioned oats
- 2 tablespoons cornstarch
- 1 teaspoon baking powder
- 1 teaspoon kosher salt
- 2 large crisp apples, peeled, cored with an apple corer, sliced into ¼"-thick rings
Special equipment:

- A deep-fry thermometer

Preparation

Step 1

In a shallow bowl, combine ½ cup sugar and 1 teaspoon cinnamon; set aside.

Step 2

Fit a thermometer to a large pot and pour in enough oil to weigh 3". Heat until a thermometer reads 375°F over medium-high heat.

Step 3

In the meantime, grind oats to a coarse powder in a food processor. In a big mixing bowl, combine rice flour, salt, baking powder, cornstarch, and the remaining 2 tbsp sugar and ½ tsp cinnamon.

Step 4

Whisk in the egg and ½ cup club soda, then gradually add more soda by the tablespoonful until the batter has the consistency of pancake batter.

Step 5

Working in batches and keeping the oil temperature steady, dip apple rings in batter and fry until golden brown and crisp, about 4 minutes.

Step 6

Place the fritters to a paper towel–lined plate; allow to drain briefly, then toss in remaining cinnamon sugar.

Gluten-Free Oat and Buckwheat Pancakes

It's delicious! Even if you don't usually like pancakes, these have a great flavor that make them more interesting than the bland white ones.

These pancakes are highly addictive: Any leftovers can be frozen and reheated by toasting them gently.

Prep Time: 15 minutes

Prep Time: 30 minutes

Servings: 20

Ingredients

- 2 cups buttermilk
- 1 cup old-fashioned oats (not quickcooking)
- 3 large eggs
- ½ cup buckwheat flour
- 1 teaspoon baking powder
- 2 tablespoons ground flaxseeds
- 1 tablespoon sugar
- 1 teaspoon baking soda
- ½ teaspoon kosher salt
- ¼ cup (½ stick) unsalted butter, plus more for pan

60

- pure maple syrup (for garnish)

Preparation

Step 1

Preheat oven to 200°. In a small saucepan over medium heat, melt ¼ cup butter and cook, stirring frequently, till butter foams, then browns (do not burn), 4–5 minutes. Let cool slightly.

Step 2

In a food processor, puree the buttermilk and oats until smooth. Combine the eggs, buckwheat flour, flaxseeds, sugar, baking powder, baking soda, and salt in a large food processor. Blend for 30 seconds on high. Blend in the butter until it is fully combined.

Step 3

Heat a large nonstick skillet over medium. Coat very gently with butter. Working in batches, spoon about 3 tablespoons of batter per pancake into skillet and cook for 3 minutes, or until bottoms are golden brown.

Step 4

In a small saucepan over medium heat, melt ¼ cup butter and cook, stirring frequently, till butter foams, then browns (do not burn), 4–5 minutes. Let cool slightly.

Step 5

In a food processor, puree the buttermilk and oats until smooth. Combine the eggs, buckwheat flour, flaxseeds, sugar, baking powder, baking soda, and salt in the food processor. Blend for 30 seconds on high. Blend in the butter until it is fully combined.

Step 6

Heat a large nonstick skillet over medium. Coat very gently with butter. Working in batches, spoon about 3 tablespoons of batter per pancake into skillet and cook for 3 minutes, or until bottoms are golden brown and tops are evenly covered in bubbles and tops are evenly covered in bubbles.

Step 7

Turn the side and cook throughout, until undersides are golden, for about 2 minutes.

Keep warm in the oven and serve with plenty of syrup.

Note: Pancakes can be made 2 weeks in advance; wrap in plastic and freeze.

Gluten-Free Pizza Crust

Prep Time: 40 minutes

Cook Time: 1 hour

Servings: 12" crusts

Ingredients

1 teaspoon instant or active dry yeast

2¼ cups gluten-free baking flour, ⅓ cup almond meal

preferably king Arthur measure for measure (about 10 ounces)

2 teaspoons sugar

3 tablespoons ground flaxseeds

1 tablespoon diamond crystal (approx. 1¾ 1 tablespoon plus 1½ teaspoons apple cider vinegar

teaspoons Morton kosher salt) 1½

teaspoons baking powder ¼ cup olive oil,

plus more for pans pizza sauce, cheese,

and herbs (for garnish)

Preparation

Step 1

In a small mixing bowl, combine the sugar and ⅓ cups warm (not hot, ideally around 100°) water. Sprinkle yeast over the top and set aside until it starts to foam and smells like bread (if it doesn't foam after 10 minutes, get fresh yeast).

Step 2

But then, in the bowl of a stand mixer fitted with the paddle attachment, whisk together flour, almond meal, flaxseeds, salt, and baking powder.

Step 3

After that, add the yeast mixture, ¼ cup oil, and vinegar. Continue to beat on medium speed for 2–3 minutes, or until the dough is smooth and sticky (it should have the consistency of cake batter).

Step 4

Seal the bowl with plastic wrap and let rise in a warm place for an hour, or until dough is slightly puffed (it will not rise as dramatically as regular dough), and poking a finger into dough shows bubbles within.

Step 5

Preheat oven to 325°. Lightly brush 2 large heatproof nonstick saucepans with oil (nonstick baking sheets, or rimmed baking sheets lined with a silpat, are better options).

Step 6

Divide the dough between the two skillets (if you only have 1 skillet, freeze the remaining dough until ready to use). Spread the dough to around ¼" thick with a large offset spatula or a rubber spatula loosely coated with oil. Cover with plastic wrap and set aside for 20–30 minutes, or until the dough has slightly puffed up again.

Step 7

Bake for 30–40 minutes, turning saucepans halfway through, until very lightly browned across the top and dough springs back.

Step 8

Place a rack in the top third of the oven and heat it up to 425°. Sauce, cheese, and herbs may be added to the crusts as needed. Bake pizzas for 10–12 minutes, or until cheese is melted and bubbling and the crust is golden brown and crunchy underneath.

BLT Chopped Salad

Prep Time: 15 minutes

Cook Time: 15 minutes

Servings: 4

Ingredients

Salad

- ½ cup corn
- 4 slices jones dairy farm dry aged bacon shredded
- ¼ cup goat cheese crumbled
- 4 cups romaine lettuce chopped
- avocado shredded
- 1 cup cherry tomatoes halved

Lime Vinaigrette

- ¼ cup olive oil
- ¼ cup apple cider vinegar

Lime zest

- 2 tablespoons lime juice
- 1 teaspoon sugar

Preparation

Step 1

Heat sizeable skillet over medium-high heat.

Step 2

Add bacon and cook until brown and crispy, about 6-8 minutes. Transfer to paper towellined plate.

Step 3

In large bowl, combine romaine lettuce, avocado, tomatoes, corn, goat cheese and bacon; set aside.

Step 4

In medium bowl, whisk together olive oil, apple cider vinegar, lime zest, lime juice, and sugar.

Step 5

Pour vinaigrette over lettuce and toss gently to coat. Serve immediately.

Nutrition Facts Per Serving

Calories 265 |**Total Fat** 27g |**Sodium** 205mg |**Total Carb.** 11g |**Sugars** 5g

Protein 6g

Gluten-Free Shells with Beets, Ricotta, and Pistachios

No joke! good gluten-free pastas exist.

Prep Time: 15 minutes

Cook Time: 20 minutes

Ingredients

- ⅓ cup raw pistachios
- Kosher salt
- 1 cup ricotta
- 1 teaspoon plus 5 tbsp. Olive oil; plus, more for drizzling
- freshly ground black pepper
- 2 pounds small golden beets, scrubbed
- 1 large shallot, diced
- Flaky sea salt
- tablespoons champagne vinegar
- 12 ounces gluten-free shells or other short pasta

- 1 tablespoon well chopped fresh chives

Preparation

Step 1

Preheat the oven to 350°. Pistachios should be toasted on a baking sheet for 8–10 minutes, stirring periodically. Allow to cool before chopping.

Step 2

Toss with 1 tsp. oil and kosher salt and pepper in a small bowl, after chopped.

Step 3

In a food processor, blend ricotta and 1 tablespoon oil until smooth (or whisk in a bowl); sprinkle with kosher salt and pepper.

Step 3

In a large pot of boiling salted water, cook beets for 12–15 minutes, or until just tender. Allow to cool slightly before transferring to a kitchen towel. Remove the skins with paper towels and cut into ¼" thick slices. Toss with shallot, vinegar, and 4 tablespoons oil in a big mixing bowl; season with kosher salt and pepper.

Step 4

Bring the beet cooking liquid back to a boil and use it to cook the pasta until al dente, stirring occasionally. Drain the pasta, reserving ½ cup of the cooking water.

Step 5

Meanwhile, heat a sizeable skillet over medium-high. Cook the beets and dressing for 8–10 minutes, tossing occasionally, until beets are golden brown in spots. Cook, tossing, add more cooking liquid as required, until pasta is thoroughly coated.

Step 6

Serve pasta with ricotta, pistachios, and chives, drizzled with olive oil. Season with salt and pepper to taste.

Casein-Free / Dairy-Free Autism Recipes

Certain behaviors in some children can be intensified by dairy products. Fortunately, there are ways to avoid dairy without compromising their wellbeing. Dairy-free products are available in many local supermarkets. Simply look through the organic products category.

However, check the labels carefully, as many products you wouldn't expect to contain dairy can contain it.

Yummy Honey Chicken Kabobs

Chicken kebab with honey and vegetables. You can soak them overnight, and then put these barbecues in an outdoor barbecue as a delicious substitute for the usual barbecue prices! You can also use fresh mushrooms and cherry tomatoes. (This can also be done in broilers.)

Prep Time: 15 minutes

Cook Time: 15 minutes

Additional: 2 hours

Servings: 12

Ingredients

- ⅓ cup honey

- ⅓ cup soy sauce
- ¼ cup vegetable oil
- ¼ teaspoon ground black pepper
- 8 skinless, boneless chicken breast halves – cut into 1-inch cubes

- small onions, finely chopped
- 2 cloves garlic
- 2 red bell peppers, finely chopped

Preparation

Step 1

Whisk together the oil, honey, soy sauce, and pepper in a big mixing bowl. Save a small amount of the marinade to brush on the kabobs as they're cooking before adding the chicken.

Step 2

Place the chicken, garlic, onions, and peppers in a bowl and marinate for at least 2 hours in the refrigerator (the longer the better).

Step 3

Preheat the grill to medium-high.

Step 4

Drain and discard the marinade from the chicken and vegetables. Place chicken and veggies conversely onto the skewers.

Step 5

Gently grease the grill with oil. Place the skewers on the grill. grill for 12 to 15 minutes, or until the chicken juices are clear. Turn frequently and brush with marinade.

<u>Nutrition Facts Per Serving</u>

Calories 175 |**Protein** 18g | **Carb.** 12.4g |**Fat** 7g |**Sodium** 442mg

Baked Honey Mustard Chicken

It's quick and easy to prepare, and kids love it too!

Prep Time: 15 mins

Cook Time: 40 minutes

Ingredients

- ½ cup honey
- 6 skinless, boneless chicken breast halves
- 1 teaspoon paprika
- 1 teaspoon salt and pepper to taste
- ½ teaspoon dried parsley
- ½ cup prepared mustard
- 1 teaspoon dried basil

Preparation

Step 1

Preheat the oven to 350 degrees F.

Step 2

Season the chicken breasts with salt and pepper and put them in a lightly greased 9x13 inch baking dish. Combine the sugar, mustard, basil, paprika, and parsley in a small cup. Mix thoroughly. Brush the chicken with ½ tablespoons of the mixture.

Step 3

Preheat the oven to 350°F and bake for 30 minutes. Brush the remaining ½ tablespoons of honey mustard mixture over the chicken bits. Bake for 10 to 15 minutes more, or until the chicken is no longer pink and the juices are clear. Let cool for 10 minutes before serving.

<u>**Nutrition Facts Per Serving**</u>

Calories 234 |**Protein** 25g | **Total Carb.** 28g | **Total Fat** 4g | **Sodium** 294mg

BBQ Pork for Sandwiches

It's easy and very tasty. Serve with buns and French fries or chips.

Prep Time: 15 minutes

Cook Time: 30 mins

Servings: 12

Ingredients

- 3 pounds boneless pork ribs
- 14-ounce can beef broth

- 18-ounce bottle barbeque sauce

Preparation

Step 1

Add boneless pork ribs to a slow cooker with a can of beef broth. Cook for few hours on high, or until meat shreds easily. Remove the meat from the pan and shred it with two forks. It will seem that it isn't acting right away, but it will eventually.

Step 2

Preheat the oven to 350 degrees F. Stir the barbeque sauce into the shredded pork in a Dutch oven or iron skillet.

Step 3

Bake for 30 minutes, or until thoroughly cooked in a preheated oven.

<u>Nutrition Facts Per Serving</u>

Calories 358 | **Protein** 32g | **Total Carb.** 15.2g | **Total Fat** 18.1g | **Sodium** 623mg

Pork and Apple Tamales

Serve as a fast dinner, brown-bag lunch, hearty snack, or even a fun appetizer with this family favorite.

Servings: 3 dozen

Prep Time: 45 minutes + soaking

Cook Time: 45 minutes

Ingredients

- 44 dried corn husks **Dough:**

- 3 cups masa harina
- 2 cups water
- teaspoon salt
- cup lard or shortening **Filling:**

- 1-pound ground pork or beef
- ½ cup well chopped onion
- 1 teaspoon sugar
- 1 garlic clove, minced

- • can (10-3/4 ounces) tomato puree
- • tart medium apple, peeled and shredded
- • ½ cup chopped almonds, toasted
- • ¼ cup minced fresh parsley
- • 1 tablespoon cider vinegar
- • ½ teaspoon ground coriander
- • 1 cup chicken broth or water
- • ½ teaspoon coarsely ground pepper
- • ½ teaspoon chili powder
- • ¼ teaspoon ground cumin

Preparation

Soak the corn husks in cold water, covered overnight.

Step 1

Mix masa harina and water to make the dough. Cover and set aside for 30 minutes. Meanwhile, beat the lard and salt together in a separate bowl until the mixture resembles beaten egg whites for about 5 minutes. Add 2 tablespoons masa harina mixture at a time, beating continuously

Step 2

 In a large skillet over medium heat, cook pork and onion, crumbling meat, until meat is no longer pink. Add garlic; cook 1 minute longer. Drain the water. Add the remaining ten ingredients. Allow the water to boil.

Step 3

Reduce heat to low and simmer for 25 minutes, covered. Allow to cool slightly.

Step 4

Drain and pat dry corn husks; tear 7-8 husks into 36 strips for binding tamales. Cover husks with plastic wrap and a damp towel until ready to use to keep them from drying out.

Step 5

Spread 2-3 tbsp. dough to within ½ inches of side edges on the wide end of each remaining husk; top with 1-2 tbsp. filling. Fold the long sides of the husk over the filling, slightly overlapping. Fold the narrow end of the husk over and secure with a husk strip.

Step 6

Place tamales upright in a big steamer basket in a 6-quart stockpot over broth. Bring to a boil, then cover and steam for 45 minutes, or until the dough peels away from the husk.

Nutrition Facts Per Serving

Calories 382 |**Total** Fat 26g |**Sodium** 308mg | **Total Carb.** 21g | **Sugar** 3g | **Fiber** 4g | **Protein** 12g

Cashew Milk

You'll will never buy ready-made cashew milk again because this is so easy and delicious! Simply strain into cheesecloth for a silkysmooth texture.

Prep Time: 10 minutes

Servings: 12 cups

Ingredients

- 3 cups raw cashews
- 10 cups water, divided
- ¼ cup honey

Preparation

Step 1

Pour enough water to cover the cashews in a bowl, about 2 cups. Refrigerate for 12 to 16 hours.

Step 2

In a high-powered blender, mix the cashews and soaking water. Add the remaining 8 cups of water, as well as the honey. Blend on high speed until absolutely smooth.

Nutrition Facts Per Serving

Calories 210 | **Protein** 6g | **Total Carb.** 15g | **Total Fat** 14g | **Sodium** 13mg

Dairy-Free Chocolate Pudding

This vegan chocolate pudding is plain, smooth, and creamy. You can choose use ground chocolate as a substitute for cocoa.

Prep Time: 10 minutes

Cook Time: 10 minutes

Additional: 25 minutes

Ingredients

- ¼ cup white sugar
- 1 ½ cups soy milk
- ¼ cup unsweetened cocoa powder
- 3 tablespoons cornstarch
- 2 tablespoons water

- ¼ teaspoon vanilla extract

Preparation

Step 1

In medium bowl, mix the cornstarch and water to form a paste.

Step 2

Stir together the soy milk, vanilla, sugar, cocoa, and cornstarch mixture in a large saucepan over medium heat. Cook until the mixture boils, stirring continuously. Cook, stirring constantly, until the mixture thickens.

Step 3

Remove the pan from the heat. When the pudding cools, it will thicken even more. **Step 4**

Allow to cool for five minutes before placing in the refrigerator to cool fully.

<u>Nutrition Facts Per Serving</u>

Calories 268 | **Protein** 7g | **Total Carb.** 53.3g | **Total** Fat 4g | **Sodium** 95mg

Cranberry Meatballs

Prep Time: 20 min.

Cook Time: 20 min.

Ingredients

- 1 cup cornflake crumbs
- 2 tablespoons soy sauce
- 2 large eggs, slightly beaten
- 2 pounds ground pork
- ½ teaspoon salt
- 1/3 cup ketchup
- 2 tablespoons dried onion, finely chopped
- tablespoon dried parsley flakes
- ¼ teaspoon pepper **Sauce:**

- 3 tablespoons brown sugar
- 1 can jellied cranberry sauce
- 1 cup ketchup
- 1 tablespoon lemon juice

Preparation

Step 1

Preheat the oven to 350 ºc. Combine the first eight ingredients in a bowl. Mix in the pork delicately but thoroughly. Form meatballs that are 1 inch in diameter.

Step 2

In a 15x10x1-in. pan, place on a greased rack. Bake meatballs for 20-25 minutes, or until a thermometer reads 160°. Drain meatballs on paper towels.

Step 3

Mix and cook the sauce ingredients in a sizeable saucepan over medium heat until well combined. Add the meatballs and heat up for 23 minutes. Serve warm.

<u>**Nutrition Facts Per Serving**</u>

Calories 60 | **Total Fat** 2g | **Sodium** 140mg | **Total Carb.** 5g | **Sugar** 4g | **Protein** 3g
Blushing Grapefruit Sorbet

This sorbet is not too sweet. Indeed, it is best choice during holidays because there are many citrus fruits present. You can also try it as a refreshing summer drink.

Prep Time: 35 minutes+ freezing

Servings: 1 quart

Ingredients

- 3 cups water
- 2 whole star anise
- 1 cup sugar
- 1 tablespoon grated grapefruit zest
- 1 tablespoon minced fresh gingerroot
- ½ cup honey
- 2 whole cloves
- bay leaf
- cups ruby red grapefruit juice, refrigerated
- tablespoons lemon juice

Preparation

Step 1

Combine the first eight ingredients in a sizeable saucepan. Bring to a boil; cook for 20 minutes or until liquid is reduced by half. Set aside to cool after straining.

Step 2

Combine the grapefruit mixture, lemon juices, as well as the sugar syrup, in a big mixing bowl. Fill ice cream freezer cylinder halfway with mixture; freeze according to manufacturer's instructions. Freeze for four hours or until solid.

Baked Pot Stickers with Dipping Sauce

Prep Time: 30 minutes

Bake: 15 minutes/batch

Servings: 4 dozen (3/4 cup sauce)

Ingredients

- 2 cups shredded cooked chicken breast
- 4 green onions, finely chopped
- ¼ cup shredded carrots
- ¼ 1 garlic clove, minced
- can (8 ounces) water chestnuts, drained and diced
- cup reduced-fat mayonnaise
- large egg white
- 1 tablespoon reduced-sodium soy sauce

- 1 teaspoon grated fresh gingerroot
- 48 wonton wrappers
- Cooking spray **Sauce**:

- ½ cup jalapeno pepper jelly
- 2 tablespoons reduced-sodium soy sauce
- ¼ cup rice vinegar

Directions

Step 1

Preheat the oven to 425°. In a large bowl, combine the first 9 ingredients.

Step 2

Place 2 teaspoons of filling in center of a wonton wrapper. (Cover rest of wrappers with a damp paper towel until ready to use.)

Step 3

Moisten wrapper edges with water. Fold edge over filling and roll to form a log; twist ends to seal. Repeat with remaining wrappers and filling. **Step 4**

Place pot stickers on a baking sheet coated with cooking spray; spritz each with cooking spray. Bake 12-15 minutes or until edges are golden brown.

Step 5

Meanwhile, place jelly in a small microwavesafe bowl; microwave, covered, on high until melted. Stir in vinegar and soy sauce. Serve sauce with pot stickers.

<u>**Nutrition Facts Per Serving**</u>

Calories 55 | **Total** Fat 1g | **Sodium** 105mg
Total Carb. 8g | **Sugar** 2g | **Protein** 3g

Carb-Free Autism Recipes

Low-carb and no-carb diets are two other common alternatives that have been tested for their effect on autistic children. The goal is to eliminate all refined carbohydrates from their diet. This involves potatoes, sugary snacks, and fruit juice. One serving of whole fruit per day is recommended for certain diets. Despite the fact that it is a very strict diet, it has many advantages, including increased concentration and energy. Both of these things can be helpful for your kids.

Sausage & Egg Breakfast Bites

Simple, fast, convenient, healthy, delicious. What more can you ask for from your breakfast?

Prep Time: 15 minutes

Cook Time: 45 minutes

Servings: 4

Ingredients:

- 9 medium eggs
- 1 cup of crumbled, uncooked sausage (homemade sausage.)
- 1 cup of dark greens (this recipe used kale, but you can use beet greens or swiss chard)
- a small bunch of parsley (about ½ cup minced)
- 2 tablespoons of primal kitchen avocado oil

Preparation

Step 1

Preheat the oven to 375 F.

Step 2

Remove the stems from kale before slicing the greens into thin strips. Over medium heat, sauté the greens for several minutes in avocado oil.

Step 3

In the same pan, add the crumbled sausage. Continue to sauté until the sausage is almost finished, then remove from the heat.

Step 4

Whisk the 9 eggs together in a mixing bowl.

Step 5

In the egg mixture, add the parsley, kale, and sausage.

Step 6

Sprinkle an 8×8 pan with avocado oil.

Step 7

Stir the egg mixture into the pan. Preheat the oven to 200°F and bake for 20-25 minutes, or until the mixture is firm and browning on top.

Step 8

Allow to cool before cutting into squares after removing the pan from the oven.

Nutrition Facts Per Serving

Calories 295 | **Total** Fat 22g | **Protein** 20g
Total Carb. 3g

Pepperoni Meatza

It's made almost exactly the same as pizza, except that it uses ground beef as the crust. Sounds funny at first, but it is perfectly delicious and very filling. This is a perfect dish to prepare ahead of time and enjoy later as leftovers.

Prep Time: 30 minutes

Cook Time: 15 minutes

Yield: 1 -12x17-inch pizza

Ingredients

- 1 tablespoon salt
- cup tomato sauce
- 1 teaspoon garlic salt
- 2 medium eggs
- teaspoon caraway seeds (optional)
- teaspoon dried oregano
- 1 teaspoon ground black pepper
- 1 (3.5 ounce) package sliced pepperoni, or to taste
- teaspoon red pepper flakes, or to taste (optional)
- 2 pounds extra lean ground beef
- ½ cup grated Parmesan cheese
- (12 ounce) package shredded mozzarella cheese

Preparation

Step 1

Preheat the oven to 450 degrees F.

Step 2

In a small bowl, combine salt, caraway seeds, oregano, garlic salt, ground black pepper, and crushed red pepper flakes.

Step 3

In a mixing bowl, thoroughly combine the ground beef and eggs. Combine the beef, Parmesan cheese, and seasoning mixture. Spread the ground beef mixture uniformly in a 12x17-inch pan.

Step 4

Bake for 10 minutes in a preheated oven until the meat is no longer pink. Grease should be removed.

Step 5

Turn on the oven's broiler and place the oven rack about 6 inches from the heat source.

Step 6

Over the cooked meat, sprinkle ⅓ of the mozzarella cheese, then an even layer of tomato sauce. Add another portion of the mozzarella cheese to the sauce and top with pepperoni slices. Stir the remaining mozzarella cheese over pizza.

Step 7

Broil for 3 to 5 minutes, or until cheese is melted, bubbling, and lightly browned.

Nutrition Facts Per Serving

Calories 500 | **Protein** 56.5g | **Total Carb.** 5g | **Total Fat** 27g | **Sodium** 220mg

Southwest Egg and Cheese Boats

The filling takes just a few minutes to put together, and the result is a flavorful hot sandwich that's perfect for a casual brunch or weeknight dinner.

Prep Time: 15 minutes

Cook Time: 30 mins

Additional: 3 mins

Servings: 2

Ingredients

- 4 eggs
- 2 oval sandwich rolls
- 1 (4 ounce) can chopped green chile peppers
- ¼ teaspoon salt
- 3 tablespoons whole milk
- cup shredded sharp Cheddar cheese
- ½ cup shredded pepper Jack cheese
- ½ teaspoon smoked paprika

Preparation

Step 1

Preheat the oven to 350 degrees F. Line up a rimmed baking sheet with parchment paper.

Step 2

Cut each roll into a V shape, leaving the ends untouched. Pull out the V-shaped wedge. To form shallow bread bowls, gently hollow out rolls, being careful not to cut through the bottom or sides. Place the bread bowls on the baking sheet that has been prepared.

Step 3

Whisk the eggs in a bowl. Whisk in the milk until it is fully mixed. Green chile peppers, Cheddar cheese, pepper Jack cheese, paprika, and salt are all added at this stage. Slowly pour the mixture into the rolls, spreading uniformly with a spoon.

Step 4

Bake for 30 minutes in a preheated oven until the egg mixture is fully set and the cheese is lightly browned. Cool for 3 minutes before serving.

<u>Nutrition Facts Per Serving</u>

Calories 574 | protein 34g | **Total Carb.** 5g **Total** fat 42g | sodium 716mg

Garlic Chicken

It's easy to make; simply dip and bake! In a breaded chicken dish, there's a touch of garlic. Delicious!

Prep Time: 15 minutes

Cook Time: 40 minutes

Ingredients

- ¼ cup olive oil
- ¼ cup Italian-seasoned bread crumbs
- 2 cloves garlic, minced
- ¼ cup grated Parmesan cheese
- ¼ cup grated Parmesan cheese
- 4 skinless, boneless chicken breast halves cup olive oil
- ¼ cup Italian-seasoned bread crumbs
- 4 skinless, boneless chicken breast halves

Preparation

Step 1

Preheat the oven to 425 degrees F (220 degrees C).

Step 2

In a small saucepan, heat the olive oil and garlic over low heat for 1 to 2 minutes. Transfer garlic and oil to a small bowl.

Step 3

In a different shallow dish, mix bread crumbs and Parmesan cheese.

Step 4

Use tongs to dip the chicken breasts in the olive oil-garlic mixture, then move to the bread crumb mixture and turn to coat evenly. Place the chicken in a shallow baking dish that has been prepared.

Step 5

Bake for 30 to 35 minutes in a preheated oven until pink and juices run clear. Insert an instant-read thermometer in the middle; it should read at least 165 degrees F (74 degrees C).

<u>**Nutrition Facts Per Serving**</u>

Calories 300 | **Protein** 33g | **Total Carb.** 5g | **Total Fat** 14g| **Cholesterol** 72mg | **Sodium** 261.2mg

Rosemary Ranch Chicken Kabobs

The chicken in this rosemary ranch recipe is so tender and juicy that it will melt in your mouth. Even the most discerning eater can beg for the last bite.

Prep Time: 50 minutes

Cook Time: 10 minutes

Servings: 6

Ingredients

- ½ cup ranch dressing
- ½ cup olive oil
- 3 tablespoons Worcestershire sauce
- ¼ teaspoon ground black pepper, for taste
- tablespoon minced fresh rosemary
- 2 teaspoons salt
- teaspoon lemon juice
- teaspoon white vinegar
- tablespoon white sugar, for taste
  (optional)
- 5 skinless, boneless chicken breast halves – sliced into 1-inch cubes

Preparation

Step 1

Combine the olive oil, ranch dressing, Worcestershire sauce, pepper, salt, lemon juice, white vinegar, rosemary, and sugar in a medium mixing bowl. Let stand for 5 minutes. Place the chicken in the bowl and toss it around in the marinade to coat it. Refrigerate (covered) for at least for 30 minutes.

Step 2

Preheat your grill to medium-high. Remove the chicken from the marinade and thread it onto skewers.

Step 3

Grease the grill grate cautiously. Grill for 8 to 10 minutes, or until the chicken is no longer pink in the center and the juices run clear.

<u>**Nutrition Facts Per Serving**</u>

Calories 373 | **Protein** 19g | **Total Carb.** 4.8g | **Total** Fat 30.7g | **Cholesterol** 59.2mg | **Sodium** 1092mg

Crustless Spinach Quiche

Serve this for brunch during summer; with a side of sausage links and a fruit bowl!

Prep Time: 20 mins

Cook Time: 30 mins

Servings: 6

Ingredients

- 5 eggs, whisked

- ¼ teaspoon salt
- 1 tablespoon vegetable oil
- (10 ounce) package frozen diced spinach, thawed and drained
- onion, finely chopped

- cups shredded Muenster cheese
- ⅛ teaspoon ground black pepper

Preparation

Step 1

Preheat the oven to 350 degrees F. Gently grease a 9-inch pie pan.

Step 2

In a large skillet, heat the oil over medium-high heat. Add the onion and fry, stirring every now and then until onions are soft. Stir in the spinach and cook until all liquid has evaporated.

Step 3

Combine eggs, cheese, salt, and pepper in a big mixing bowl. Stir in the spinach mixture until it is well mixed. Scoop into the pie pan that has been prepared.

Step 4

Bake for 30 minutes in a preheated oven until the eggs have set. Allow for 10 minutes to cool before serving.

<u>**Nutrition Facts Per Serving**</u>

Calories 311 | **Protein** 21g | **Total Carb.** 4.8g | **Total** Fat 23g | **Cholesterol** 209mg | **Sodium** 545.6mg

Cheesy Garlic Bread

Prep Time: 15 minutes

Cook Time: 25 minutes

Yield: 10

Ingredients

Bread Base

- 3 egg whites, roughly whisked
- ¼ cup warm water
- ¼ cup almond flour (I use Well bee's)
- tablespoon coconut flour
- 1 tsp. coconut sugar
- 1 tsp. live yeast granules
- 2 tablespoon olive oil or avocado oil
- ½ cup shredded mozzarella cheese
- ¼ tsp. salt
- 2 tsp. baking powder
- ¼ tsp. garlic powder
- ½ tsp. xanthan or guar gum (optional)

Topping

- ¼ tsp. salt
- 2 tablespoon butter, melted
- ¼ tsp. garlic powder
- ½ tsp. Italian seasoning
- 1 cup shredded mozzarella cheese

Preparation

Step 1

Preheat the oven to 400 degrees.

Step 2

Combine the almond and coconut flours, salt, baking powder, garlic powder, and xanthan gum in a big mixing bowl. Stir all together thoroughly.

Step 3

Combine the warm water and sugar in a small cup or bowl and stir until sugar is dissolved, then add yeast. Set aside for a few minutes.

Step 4

Add the olive oil and yeast-water mixture to the flour mixture and stir well with a rubber spatula. Pour the in beaten eggs and continue to mix.

Step 5

Mix in the ½ cup mozzarella shreds with a spatula until a pleasant dough forms and the cheese is uniformly dispersed.

Step 6

Grease a 9-by-9-inch square cake pan or a large baking sheet with butter. Fill a cake pan or baking sheet halfway with batter. If you're freeforming the dough on a cookie sheet, shape it into a rectangle or square.

Step 7

Bake for 15-17 minutes at 400 degrees, or until the sides of the crust are golden brown. Remove the top and discard.

Step 8

Combine butter, garlic powder, and salt in a small cup. Brush over the top of the garlic bread base after thoroughly mixing. Make sure the butter is all over the spot!

Step 9

Sprinkle shredded mozzarella cheese on top of the bread, then dress with Italian seasoning.

Step 10

Bake for 10 minutes at 400 degrees, or until cheese is melted. Turn on the broiler for the last 3 minutes to brown the cheese.

Step 11

 Remove the bread from the oven and set it aside for 5-12 minutes before serving.

Nutrition Facts Per Serving

Calories 177 | **Total Carb.** 4g | **Fiber** 2g | **Total Fat** 15g | **Protein** 8g

Bacon-Wrapped Mini Meatloaves

For years, these mini bacon-wrapped meatloaves have been a crowd-pleaser, and no one has ever turned them down. The mini meatloaves are also very simple to make. They don't take long to prepare and are ready in the oven in no time.

Prep Time: 20 minutes

Cook Time: 30 minutes

Servings:

Ingredients

- ½ lb. bacon, sliced in small chunks
- ¼ cup coconut milk
- 1 lb. ground beef
- 8 additional strips of bacon;
- Fresh parsley, finely chopped
- 2 garlic cloves, minced
- 1/3 cup fresh chives, diced
- Freshly ground black pepper for taste

Preparation

Step 1

Preheat the oven to 400 F.

Step 2

Combine the ground beef, bacon bits, garlic, chives, and coconut milk in large mixing bowl. In the large mixing bowl, combine all of the ingredients until they are well combined. To save time, you can use an electric mixer.

Step 3

Toss in a pinch of freshly ground black pepper and season to taste. There's no need to salt the mixture because the bacon is salty enough.

Step 4

Place a slice of bacon around the sides of each hole in a medium muffin pan.

Step 5

Fill the remaining eight holes in the same way with the beef mixture.

Step 6

Preheat the oven to 350°F and bake for 30 minutes.

Step 7

Remove the mini meatloaves from the muffin tin once they are cool enough to handle and serve with fresh parsley on top.

Mushroom Pork Chops

It's fast, simple and very tasty. Served over brown rice; one of my family's favorites.

Prep Time: 10 mins

Cook Time: 30 mins

Servings: 4

Yield: 4

Ingredients

- 1 pinch garlic salt to taste
- 1 onion, finely chopped
- ½ pound fresh mushrooms, finely chopped
- salt and pepper to taste
- 4 pork chops
- can condensed cream of mushroom soup

Preparation

Step 1

Season the pork chops with salt, pepper, and garlic salt.

Step 2

Brown the chops in a large skillet over mediumhigh heat. Sauté for one minute with the onion and mushrooms. Pour mushroom soup over the chops.

Step 3

Reduce the heat to medium-low and cover the skillet. Cook for 20 to 30 minutes, or until chops are ready.

<u>**Nutrition Facts Per Serving**</u>

Calories 211 | **Protein** 26g | **Total Carb.** 6g **Total Fat** 7g | **Cholesterol** 64.9mg | **Sodium** 924mg

D's Famous Salsa

Prep Time: 10 mins

Servings: 16

Ingredients

- 2 (14.5 ounce) cans stewed tomatoes
- 1 teaspoon salt
- ½ onion, finely chopped
- 1 teaspoon crushed garlic
- ½ lime, juiced
- ¼ cup canned sliced green chiles, to taste
- 3 tablespoons chopped fresh cilantro

Directions

Step 1

In a blender or food processor, combine the tomatoes, onion, garlic, lime juice, salt, green chiles, and cilantro. Blend on low until the desired consistency is reached

Sugar-Free Autism Recipes

Sugar-free recipes are another collection of recipes that are in high demand. That's understandable, given that sugar consumption contributes to many of today's health issues. We all know how tough it is to stay away from sugar because of its addictive properties. Furthermore, the fact that many children's snacks are high in sugar does not help matters.

So, here are some sugar-free alternatives to help you break the habit!

Sugar- free Apple Pie

My aunt would bake this pie for my 99-year-old diabetic grandma. She died few years ago.

Prep Time: 15 minutes

Cook Time: 45 minutes

Servings: 8

Ingredients

- 3 tablespoons cornstarch
- 1 tablespoon ground cinnamon
- 2 ounces unsweetened apple juice concentrate
- 6 cups apples, thinly sliced

Preparation

Step 1

Preheat the oven to 350 degrees F.

Step 2

Combine the cornstarch, cinnamon, and 14 cup apple juice in a mixing bowl.

Step 3

Steam the apples in the remaining apple juice in a saucepan over medium heat until soft. Stir in the cornstarch mixture until it thickens.

Step 4

Spill into bottom crust and cover with top crust. Bake 45 minutes in the oven.

<u>**Nutrition Facts Per Serving**</u>

Calories 301 | **Protein** 4g | **Total Carb.** 41g | **Total Fat** 14g | **Sodium** 235mg

Sugar-Free French Toast Casserole

Sugar and butter aren't used in this lighter version of French toast casserole, but it still tastes delicious. Make it the night before and pop it in the oven first thing in the morning for a hassle-free breakfast and brunch!

Prep Time: 15 minutes

Cook Time: 30 minutes

Additional: 10 minutes

Servings: 6

Ingredients

- Serving cooking spray (such as Pam®)
- 5 medium eggs
- 5 cups cubed bread
- 1 ½ cups milk
- 2 teaspoons ground cinnamon, divided
- 1 teaspoon vanilla extract
- ¼ cup granular sucralose sweetener (such as Splenda®), divided

Preparation

Step 1

Preheat the oven to 350 degrees F. Spray a 9x13inch baking dish with cooking spray.

Step 2

Line bottom of baking dish with bread cubes. In a mixing bowl, whisk together eggs, milk, 2 tbsp sweetener, 1 teaspoon cinnamon, and vanilla extract; pour over bread cubes. Let stand 12 minutes (or refrigerate up to overnight if desired).

Step 3

Sprinkle the remaining 2 tsp sweetener over the casserole, along with the remaining 1 tsp cinnamon.

Step 4

Bake for 25 to 35 minutes in a preheated oven, or until the casserole is set and the topping is crunchy.

<u>**Nutrition Facts Per Serving**</u>

Calories 164 | **Protein** 8g | **Total Carb.** 15g
Total Fat 5g | **Cholesterol** 128mg | **Sodium**
274mg

Sugarless Fruitcake

This moist fruitcake incorporates artificial sweetener instead of sugar and contains pineapple, musts, cranberries, and coconut.

Prep Time: 15 minutes

Cook Time: 40 minutes

Yield: 1 – 9-inch loaf cake

Ingredients

- 1 ½ cup walnuts, crushed
- 1 cup golden raisins, finely chopped
- ½ teaspoon salt
- 1 cup cranberries, finely chopped
- 1 cup unsweetened crushed pineapple
- ¼ cup grated lemon peel

- 1 cup flaked coconut
- ⅓ cup orange juice
- 8 packets artificial sweetener
- 1 teaspoon ground mace
- 1 teaspoon ground allspice
- 1 teaspoon baking soda
- 1 ½ cups all-purpose flour

Preparation

Step 1

Combine the sugar substitute and the orange juice in a mixing bowl. Pour over the cranberries that have been chopped. Soak for 1 hour, stirring often.

In a large mixing bowl, toss together the raisins, almonds, coconut, and lemon rind until well coated. Combine the cranberries and orange juice.

Step 2

Mix in the baking soda with the rest of the ingredients. Spices should be added last. Add the crushed pineapple and combine well. Fill a

greased and floured 9-inch loaf pan halfway
with batter.

Step 3

Preheat oven to 325°F (165°C) and bake for 40
minutes. Cool and serve.

Sugar-Free Peanut Butter Cookies

Prep Time: 10 minutes

Cook Time: 8 minutes

Yield: 24 cookies

Ingredients

- 2 cups smooth natural peanut butter
- 3 large eggs
- 2 cups granular no-calorie sucralose
  sweetener (e.g., Splenda ®)

Preparation

Step 1

Preheat the oven to 350 degrees F (175 degrees C). Gently grease the baking sheet.

Step 2

In a mixing bowl, thoroughly combine the peanut butter, sucralose, and eggs. Drop some spoonful of the mixture onto the baking sheet that has been prepared.

Step 3

Bake for 8 minutes in a preheated oven, or until the center appears dry.

<u>**Nutrition Facts Per Serving**</u>

Calories 140 | **Protein** 6g | **Total Carb.** 4.9g | **Total Fat** 10g | **Cholesterol** 15mg | **Sodium** 65mg

Slow Cooker Ham and Beans

This recipe is ideal for those wet and windy days when you don't have much time to cook but still want to feed your family a great meal. It's an easy, nutrient-dense meal that everyone can enjoy!

Prep Time: 10 minutes + soaking time

Cook Time: 12 hours

Servings: 8

Ingredient

1-pound dried great Northern beans, soaked overnight

- 1 tablespoon onion powder
- chicken broth
- ½ pound cooked ham, minced
- ½ teaspoon garlic salt
- dried thyme
- ½ teaspoon black pepper
- 1 tablespoon dried parsley
- ¼ teaspoon cayenne pepper

Preparation

Step 1

Rinse the beans under cold water in a colander.

Step 2

Add the beans, ham, dried thyme, chicken broth, onion powder, parsley, garlic salt, black pepper, and cayenne pepper.

Step 3

Fill the slow cooker with enough water to cover the mixture by around 2 inches. Reduce to low and simmer for 5-7 hours, stirring occasionally.

-

Step 4

After the cooking time has elapsed, stir in the ham flavor packet. If needed, season with salt. Serve, enjoy!

Nutrition Facts Per Serving

Calories 317 | **Protein** 18g | **Total Carb.** 49.8g | **Total Fat** 6g | **Cholesterol** 16mg | **Sodium** 492.5mg

Sugar Free Peanut Butter Cheesecake Ice Cream

Sugar-free ice cream is homemade with just a few ingredients and easy enough for a child to make! It's Keto-friendly, low-carb, and dairyfree.

Prep Time: 20 minutes

Servings: 8

Ingredients

- 2 cups Almond Milk unsweetened
- 1 cup peanut butter unsweetened

  8 ounces cream cheese
- ½ cup Swerve Confectioners sweetener
- 1 teaspoon vanilla extract
- 1 teaspoon toffee flavored liquid stevia or vanilla stevia

Preparation

Step 1

In a high-powered blender, mix all of the ingredients. Blend until it is well incorporated. Taste and adjust sweetener if desired.

Step 2

Fill an ice cream machine halfway with the mixture and process according to the manufacturer's instructions.

Step 3

Freeze for 1 hour or until hard enough to scoop in an airtight jar. Top with peanuts if needed!

•

No Bake Sugar Free Coffee Cheesecake (Keto, Nut Free)

This sugar-free coffee cheesecake is prepared with a gluten-free and nut-free pie crust which is keto and sugar-free all the way down to the chocolate syrup on top!

Prep Time: 20 minutes

Servings: 12

Ingredients

Crust

- ¼ cup unsweetened cocoa powder unsweetened
- ¾ cup unsweetened shredded coconut unsweetened
- ¼ tsp salt
- ½ cup sunflower seeds unsalted raw
- ¼ cup Swerve sweetener • 4 tbsp butter room temp.

Filling

- ¾ cup coffee hot
- 2½ teaspoons gelatin

- ¼ tsp salt
- 16 ounces cream cheese room temp.
- 2 tsp coffee extract

  2 tsp vanilla liquid stevia
- cup heavy whipping cream

Topping

- 1 tbsp coconut oil
- 2 ounces 85 % dark chocolate

Preparation

Step 1

Blend the coconut and sunflower seeds in a food processor until finely ground.

Step 2

In a food processor, combine the remaining crust ingredients and process until smooth.

Step 3

With your fingertips, press the crust mixture into the bottom of an 8-inch spring shape plate. Set aside. Fill a bowl or cup halfway with hot brewed coffee.

•

Step 4

Stir in the gelatin until it is fully dissolved. Set down to come to room temperature.

Step 5

Pour in the heavy whipping cream and blend on high for 5 minutes, or until the mixture looks blended and thickened.

Pour into the pan's crust. Refrigerate for at least 4 hours or overnight.

Step 6

When ready to serve, melt the chocolate and coconut oil together in a small microwave-safe bowl for 30 seconds, stirring until smooth, then pour over the cheesecake.

<u>Nutrition Facts Per Serving</u>

Calories 397 | **Total Fat** 30g | **Cholesterol** 51mg | **Sodium** 253mg | **Potassium** 155mg| **Total Carb.** 6g | **Fiber** 2g | **Sugar** 1g | **Protein** 5g | **Vitamin A** 625IU | **Calcium** 46mg

Sugar Free No Bake Raspberry Cheesecake Bites

They are best for special occasions like Valentine's Day, they're made low carb, sugar free, gluten free, and the loveliest of candies!

Prep Time: 15 minutes

Servings: 40 cheesecake bites

Ingredients

- 1 teaspoons salt
- 2 tablespoons heavy cream
- ½ cup Swerve sweetener Confectioners
- teaspoons raspberry extract
- teaspoon vanilla liquid stevia
- 8 ounces cream cheese softened
- Little drops of natural red food coloring
- ¼ cup coconut oil, melted
- 10 ounces Lily's sugar free chocolate chips melted

Preparation

Step 1

Mix the cream cheese and Swerve together in a stand mixer until smooth.

Step 2

Mix the milk, stevia, salt, raspberry extract, and natural food coloring in the food processor or blender.

Step 3

Slowly drizzle in the coconut oil and blend on high until completely combined. Scrape down the sides of the bowl to make sure it is well combined.

Step 4

Scoop batter onto a parchment-lined baking sheet using a 1- 14-inch mini pastry scoop. Makes about 40 balls.

Step 5

Refrigerate the balls for 1 hour before coating with melted chocolate.

Step 6

Coat one cheesecake bite at a time into the melted chocolate and put on a parchment-lined baking sheet. Refrigerate for at least an hour more, until ready to serve.

<u>**Nutrition Facts Per Serving**</u>

Calories 66 | **Fat** 5g | **Cholesterol** 6mg |
Sodium 18mg | **Potassium** 8mg |
Carbohydrates 1g | **Sugar** 1g | **Protein** 1g |
Calcium 6mg | **Iron** 1mg

Whole Grain Healthy Banana Bread

This banana bread is flavorful and moist. The added benefits include whole grains, high fiber, and low fat and sugar. My family eats it a lot! This recipe can also be baked in four mini loaf pans at the same temperature for 25 to 30 minutes.

Prep Time: 15 minutes

Cook Time: 1 hour

Servings: 10

Ingredients

- ½ teaspoon salt
- ¼ cup skim milk

- ¾ cup flax seed meal
- ¾ cup SPLENDA® Sugar Blend
- 6 ripe bananas, mashed
- ¼ cup low-fat sour cream
- 2 teaspoons egg whites
- 2 cups whole wheat flour
- 1 teaspoon baking soda

Preparation

Step 1

Preheat the oven to 350 degrees F (175 degrees C). Gently grease a 9x5 inch loaf pan.

Step 2

Mix together the sugar blend, flax meal, bananas, milk, sour cream, and egg whites in a medium mixing bowl until well combined. Combine the flour, baking soda, and salt in the mixing bowl; whisk in the banana mixture together until moistened. Pour into the loaf pan that has been set.

Step 3

In a preheated oven, bake for 1 hour and 10 minutes, or until a toothpick pressed into the loaf's crown comes out clean.

<u>**Nutrition Facts Per Serving**</u>

Calories 267 | **Protein** 5g | Total **Carb.** 45g | **Total Fat** 5g | **Cholesterol** 2.5mg | **Sodium** 253mg

<u>**Last Thoughts**</u>

These are just a few recipes to get you started. As you might be aware, sticking to a diet is a lifestyle change. And any diet would require a certain amount of trial and error. Expect certain stuff to not go as planned at first. But don't let your enthusiasm be stifled by discouragement. Recognize that setbacks are a normal part of the method.

Find inspiration wherever you can. Making meal planning a collaborative task is one concept. Allow your child to assist you in preparing the meal. Make them go to the grocery store and look for the products. Enable them to weigh the ingredients. As a consequence, they become a part of the process. This will aid in building of a relationship based on the food experience.

www.ingramcontent.com/pod-product-compliance
Lightning Source LLC
Chambersburg PA
CBHW070126260726
48658CB00001B/284